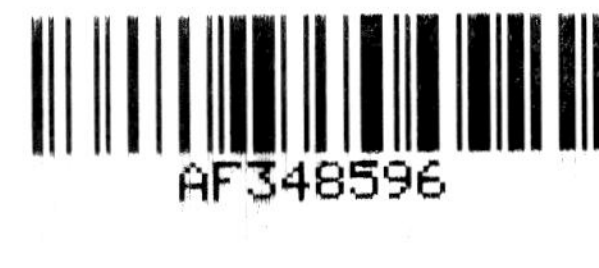
AF348596

Made in the USA
Monee, IL
07 July 2026

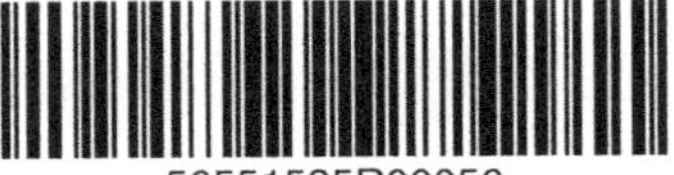

56551535R00056